▼▲▼

The Healer

Compiled by
J. Stephen Hines

Forward Movement Publications
Cincinnati, Ohio

©1998
Forward Movement Publications
412 Sycamore Street
Cincinnati, Ohio 45202

John Stephen Hines
is the rector of
St. Luke's Episcopal Church,
Asheville, North Carolina

Contents

Introduction

I am a great fan of stories, stories not only catch and keep my attention, they also touch me in places that other literary genre (like phone books and IRS forms and even some sermons I have heard or read!) do not. They touch my imagination and, at their best, my heart. Why is this? If pushed, I guess I would say that good stories are "sacramental". The tried and true definition still holds, "an outward and visible sign of an inward and spiritual grace". The outward and visible signs are the ink and the paper. The inward and spiritual grace is the miraculous ability of words on a piece of paper to transport us into a different psychological or spiritual realm and, in the case of the stories in this book, into the Kingdom of God, that place deep down in our selves where we understand that God is love and that we—all of us—are bound together by God's love. That is what these stories do for me. Needless to say, I hope they will have the same effect on you.

Because I often use stories in sermons I am always on the lookout for more material and sometimes, in my more anxious moments, I worry that the supply of good stories will run out. Then I think, no, the supply will never run out. As long as there are men and women in the world (and it seems that there always have been and will continue to be) who continue to love Jesus more than their own selves, there will be others around to tell these peoples' stories.

With this in mind let me make a suggestion. Think about your favorite story or stories, stories which especially touch your soul. Write them down and send them to Forward Movement. Perhaps they will publish another collection. And then I will be able to enjoy your favorite stories as I hope you will enjoy mine.

The Rev. J. Stephen Hines

The Healer

In 1944, as a paratrooper with the legendary 101st Airborne Division, Gus Bernardoni bailed out of a plane over Holland in what turned out to be anything but a routine jump. His chute became entangled with a bundle of supplies that had also been dropped from the aircraft, forcing him into a virtual free fall for the final 300 feet of his descent onto a hostile chunk of Dutch territory. Plummeting toward earth, he had what he describes as "talk with God," during which he asked Him to bless all the friends and loved ones he would never see again. Instantaneously, Bernardoni's body went limp as wet newsprint. He survived—and, understandably, became a lifelong Christian. But for 78 days on the front line, trapped under heavy fire, Bernardoni went without proper medical treatment, his spine twisted and his right leg paralyzed.

After corrective spinal surgery restored movement to the young paratrooper's lower body, doctors at the Mayo Clinic suggested Gus swing golf clubs as part of his recuperative therapy. Employing all the tenets of a "correct" stroke—stiff left arm, head down, hips rotated, etc.—Bernardoni suffered excruciating pain. But he didn't quit. Bernardoni tells them he could have lain in a V.A. hospital and collected a pension, or convalesced at home. Or done nothing. Instead, he taught himself to play golf—not traditionally, but well. In 1974, still enduring chronic back pain 30 years after his parachuting mishap, he won the Illinois PGA Senior Championship. In 1978 he wrote a book, *Golf God's Way*, outlining his peculiarly effective methods. Now 75, Bernardoni still plays out of the Pine Meadows Golf Club in Mundelein, Illinois, north of Chicago, and coaches several Senior PGA TOUR players. But much of Bernardoni's life is devoted to work with the Special Olympics and hospitals around the country, coaching people with debilitating illnesses like multiple sclerosis, muscular dystrophy and arthritis to develop self-esteem, confidence and willpower through a game that normally inspires none of those qualities in its practitioners.

The golfers at this instructional clinic, sponsored by United Cerebral Palsy, are not looking to shave strokes off their score. They're not trying to cure a troublesome slice. They don't want to play golf *better*—they just want to play golf.

Bernardoni tells his audience that golf is really a lot simpler than most people think. "You've got to get balanced, you have to swing the club, and you have to hit the ball. That's all." To demonstrate, he hits golf balls from one foot, on his knees and facing backward. And when I say "hits," I don't mean "makes contact with." I mean *powders*.

He calls up John Irwin, who since a massive stroke, can only move his left side. He has Irwin tuck his right hand into a pocket. "Get that thing out of the way," he says. Then he adjusts Irwin's left-hand grip, turning all of his knuckles on top of the club. Shifting Irwin's torso closer to the target line to "redefine his center of gravity," Bernardoni asks his student to pick up the club and chop at the ball while exclaiming "Pow!" at impact.

"Pow, . . ." Irwin whispers, as the ball dribbles off the tee. The teacher stands with his hands on hips, in mock disbelief. Not "pow," Bernardoni says weakly. "POW!!"

His student laughs. But now he's all business. After a few emphatic practice swings, Irwin addresses his ball, makes a mighty wallop and says, "POW!!" The ball sails into the distance.

Everyone applauds heartily. But Irwin doesn't notice. Holding his golf club out like a sword, he's too busy savoring every wondrous yard of the ball's flight, a journey that he, a massive stroke victim, authored. When the ball finally comes to rest many yards from where it started, Irwin shuffles, six inches per step, over to his chair. For the remainder of the morning, that golf club never leaves his hand.

Eric Black, 11, has spina bifida. From his chest down he has no sensation, and he must be strapped into a chair. His pal Mark DeDecker, 12, has cerebral palsy and epilepsy and is deaf in one ear. Like most young boys, these two love to watch sports on television, especially Mark, whose mom says he is crazy for golf. Mark dreams, as we all do, of one day making slam dunks like Michael Jordan or hitting home runs like Ken Griffey Jr. or blasting drives like Phil Mickelson. But they are dreams that will come true only in his imagination.

Mark DeDecker and Eric Black can only watch the Masters broadcast every year. They will never play golf at Augusta National. They will never know the thrill of making par on a championship golf course.

That is why, after a dozen earnest whiffs and much cajoling, coaching and encouragement from Bernardoni, when DeDecker makes a bold one-handed swing with his 9-iron and sends his ball airborne, flying free and clear from all his earthly despairs, I am not the only one watching who has a tear in his eye. With a shot of maybe 45 yards, Mark DeDecker has just eagled the "Amen Corner" of his dreams.

"The Healer" was originally published in the May 1997 issue of *Sky*, permission to reprint from Delta Air Lines.

Transported Into The Kingdom

The Rev. Anne K. Bartlett

The record shows Our Lord ate out a lot, and every time he did, he seems to have upset the righteous and offended the pious, scandalizing them with his radical hospitality of inclusivity. Such hospitality invariably created gatherings of people who otherwise never would have associated with each other, gatherings that glimmered with the reflected light of the kingdom.

I daresay we modern-day "apossibles" have experienced such graced gatherings around Our Lord's table. They are unforgettable. The most vivid glimpse of kingdom community in my life, so far, happened a number of years ago on a New Year's Day. My nusband and I were in New York City on a brief holiday, and we wanted to begin the new year with worship. Our hotel was close by St. Bartholomew's Church on Park Avenue, which had a New Year's Day service of Holy Eucharist in the side chapel.

We walked (rather virtuously as I recall) through the streets of the sleepy, hungover city. The day was cold, the sky brilliantly clear. At the door of the chapel we were greeted by a distinguished-looking older man dressed in a double-breasted blue blazer, adorned with gold anchor buttons. Later, when Bill and I debriefed the extraordinary experience, we nicknamed him "The Commodore." The Commodore's wife was present as well, doing her practiced "gracious hostess" routine.

There were only a dozen or so of us scattered through the small chapel. I remember a pair of women, middle-aged, plain-faced, dressed in browns. A young woman with long dark hair, kneeling in the second pew, Gospel side. In front of us a couple in their thirties, the man with a backpack. An ordinary-looking priest entered from the side sanctuary door and the liturgy began.

About the time of the Gospel reading, a street person soft-shoed his way down the side aisle and staked out a standing position against the wall. A man in his sixties, I suppose, or maybe forties, it was hard to tell. Unkempt, of course, layers of raggedy clothes, eyes too bright for this world. He tried hard to contain himself, to be "appropriate," as they say. By the time we got to the prayers of the people, Bill poked me in the arm and gestured to the floor of the pew in front of us. I looked, and there was a dog, a Golden Retriever, calmly lying on the floor. His master reached into his backpack and withdrew a large book, which he proceeded to open and read with his fingers: the Book of Common Prayer, in Braille. I then noticed his companion had a white cane laid on the pew.

When we all got up to go to the altar rail to be fed with the holy food and drink of new and unending life, the beautiful dog led the way. This sight was too much for the street person, who lost his shaky control and began speaking in tongues that no one there had the gift of interpreting. Or maybe we did. Maybe we all did, because it didn't matter, we had been transported into the kingdom and it was just right that we were together, that odd little group of strangers, disciples of Jesus, children of Abraham and Sarah, at table with Our Lord, kneeling at that rail, hands outstretched. The dog lay down and put his lovely head on the needlepointed cushions. The priest blessed him.

Telling the Story

The Rev. Dr. Daniel P. Matthews

There is an old gospel hymn which goes "I Love to Tell the Story of Jesus and His Glory." The hymn reminds me of an incident which happened to me a few years ago.

When I was in college, I joined a fraternity and during the first part of my freshman year as a pledge we had to go into the chapter room every Monday night. I'll never forget. We would sit down in the chapter room as pledges and listen to a lecture by one of the "actives," one of the older guys. One active would talk about our involvement in sports, for example. And then they would hold up all the trophies and tell us who had won them and when. Then the next week it might be an active in the student government. And he would talk about what the fraternity had done in student government and what it stood for. And it kind of encouraged the young pledges, got them all enthused and excited. It was one of those things that we all sort of laughed about, but it was about the history of that chapter. It was the way we told the story about ourselves.

And we do it in our families, don't we, especially when the family gathers together and the grandchildren come and you're sitting on the porch and you say, you know, this house was built by your great-grandfather. We love to tell who we are.

I went back a few years ago to my college which I hadn't visited in many years. I went back to the fraternity house. There were some students sitting there studying. I said something to them about being an old graduate of the college and that I was a member of their fraternity 30 years ago and tried to give one of them the grip. He didn't do anything so I gave it to him again. He said, "That's not the grip." And I said, "What do you mean that isn't the Sigma Nu grip?" and he said, "This is the Phi Delta Theta house." I said, "What happened to the Sigma Nu's?" He said, "Oh, they got kicked off campus about ten years ago."

A few days later, I ran into one of my old buddies from college who had been active in the fraternity. I asked him what happened to the Sigma Nu's. He said that they got rowdy and described some events that took place and they just kicked them off campus. And, then in an amusing kind of way, he said, "You know, Dan, you remember the Monday nights we used to have where we'd sit at the feet of the old brothers and listen to the traditions of the fraternity? You know, they did away with that. I wonder if that had anything to do with the fraternity falling apart." Of course it did. They stopped telling their story.

All of us are hungry for something, yearning for something deeper than the *things* we've got. We're hungry for that "old, old story" mentioned in the gospel hymn so that we can know again what it is that we really are living for and giving our life to. Loving God and loving each other the way God loves, us, that's all. It's kind of simple but so hard to live out in an age and a culture and a time as materialistic as the one we live in right now. That is why it is so important for us to continue to tell, and retell, again and again and again, the old, old story.

Evangelism, Terrorism or Invitation?

The Rt. Rev. William Frey

A psychiatrist came to see me when I was bishop of Colorado. It's unusual for a psychiatrist to see the bishop. It's usually the other way around.

He had just moved to Colorado and came to complain about the parishes in my diocese. I asked where he had gone to church and he ticked off five or six parishes, saying that not one had the good liturgy or inspiring preaching he was used to.

I thought they were all good congregations, and in desperation I asked him to tell me about his relationship with God so that I could recommend an appropriate parish. "I was brought up in the Episcopal Church, went through Sunday school, was an acolyte, served as lay reader, vestry member, even senior warden," he said.

"That's great," I said. "You've told me about your relationship with the church. Now tell me about your relationship with God." He responded somewhat impatiently. "Well, I told you. I was brought up in the church, went . . . "

He stopped and looked at me and said, "I'm evading your question. Why am I doing that?" I said, "You're the shrink. You tell me." And he said, "I don't think I have a relationship with God. In fact, I'm not even sure God exists. What do I do?"

I asked him, as a man of science, to try a scientific experiment. "Assume that God exists and pray as if God exists," I told him. "And pray something like this: God, if you are there, reveal yourself to me. Show yourself to me in a way that I can understand and know that it's you."

"In the meantime," I continued, "frequent all those places where God is known to hang out. Keep going to church. And read the book in which so many other people have heard him speak." He thought that was a reasonably scientific way to test the gospel, and off he went.

Six months later, he brushed past my secretary, burst into my office and shouted, "It's happened!" He had come to tell me that he had come to know the Lord.

He had sought to enter into a relationship with God. He had put himself into a position to enter into a relationship with God and eventually he had entered into a personal and meaningful relationship with God, which is to say, he had begun to fulfill his vocation as a Christian.

On Passing the Peace

The Rev. Talbot James Bethell

The Kiss of Peace in the Holy Eucharist is perhaps the most misunderstood and misused (and least instructed by the clergy) aspect of the Liturgy. So many Episcopalians use the Peace as an opportunity to say "hi" to their neighbors in the pews. In many parishes the Peace has become a hug-in, or Howdy Doody Time! One hears such comments as "How are you?" "Good morning!" "Hello!", etc.

I believe the Kiss of Peace is prayer. It is the Peace of God in me greeting the Peace of God in you. The Peace is strategically placed at the conclusion of the liturgy of the word (scripture readings, sermon, creed, prayers for the people, confession, absolution, peace). We hear God's word, pray for ourselves and for the world, receive His forgiveness for our sin, and then we exchange Christ's presence in each of us, prior to our moving to the next part of the service, the liturgy of the table where we are fed sacramentally.

The most personal and powerful experience I have *ever* had in exchanging the Peace came about six years ago, when the Most Rev. Michael Ramsey, the 100th Archbishop of Canterbury (retired), visited St. David's Church, Topeka. One could see this man was praying deeply when the congregation passed the Peace. When I exchanged the Peace with him, he took my hand and repeated over and over, "The Peace of the Lord be with you. The Peace of the Lord be with you."

I felt the Lord's Peace pass into me, and literally my spirit began to dance! It was an experience I shall *never* forget. At that moment I suddenly understood the Peace. It is not *my* peace, I pass, but God's Peace. If you and I are to receive Christ in the Sacrament, we must first acknowledge God's presence in us. In doing so, we then fully commune with God at the altar.

I know many Episcopalians have difficulty with the Peace. If you are one who does, let it become a prayer for you. Pass the Christ in you to someone else, and see if Christ's Peace is returned to you! May the Peace of God which passes all understanding be always with you.

Christos Aneste, Alethos Aneste, Alleluia!

The Rev. Petroula K. Ruehlen

It was a bright, sunshiny morning, and I smiled with delight as I stepped on the colors of the stained glass window splashed on the chancel floor. I picked up the chalice and approached the row of kneeling figures at the altar rail. My first Easter Sunday as a deacon—the first woman clergy in my diocese. I went down the row, holding the very life of Christ in my hands, and, as I offered it to each expectant face, time was suspended.

And then it happened—the upturned face of the little old man, the smiling eyes sparkling with a knowing gleam, *"Christos Aneste,"* he said, Christ is Risen. His eyes kept smiling, and suddenly it was as though there were just the two of us in that vast space, the little old Lebanese man and the new woman deacon with the accent, just the two of us sharing a secret, a secret more powerful and more important than even death. "*Alethos Aneste*, He is truly Risen," came out the answer from my mouth without my even knowing it.

It was a greeting from the past, a greeting from another life, a greeting from childhood Easters in Greece. And in that moment of eternal time, it all came back. Again I was walking in the dark quiet streets a little before midnight, my short footsteps hurrying next to my father's heavier step and my mother's measured stride. I was holding my white Easter candle and a blood-red egg. Soon there were others, all converging to the center, as though all life were drawn to what was the focus of the universe that night. By the time we arrived, the church, the courtyard, even the surrounding streets were full, and people were leaning over from the balconies of apartments. The night air was full of Byzantine chant broadcast through the loudspeakers. We were waiting patiently for the *new light*. Not too much longer. "It's getting time for the Resurrection," people assured one another.

Like a wave surging from the center of the dark church, the sound reverberated through the standing crowd. *"Christos Aneste." "Alethos Aneste."* Sirens, firecrackers, ship horns from the harbor, and sometimes gun salutes exploded through the dark night. There were hugs and smiles. And we waited for the light/candle to candle/for the light of the world to come to us—holy light for each one of us to take home. We walked home silently, reverently, each one holding his candle and shielding the precious flame from the rising wind. If by any chance a sudden gust put our candles out, then we had to search for another family to give us light. Maybe in some subliminal way even then I understood what a tremendous parable that gesture was— walking in the dark streets looking for a stranger who would give the light of Christ to me.

And then came the moment I had waited for all year long. I did not know why it was so important, but my heart raced as we approached home. My father stepped ahead. He unlocked the door. And then he raised his candle high, and he carefully marked the top of the lintel with a sooty cross. *"Christos Aneste,"* he would say, *"Alethos Aneste."* And we would reverently walk into the house behind him. I can still see my mother turn into the bedroom to light the votive light before the icon of Mary and the Christ child that stood on top of her dresser. I smiled with secret pleasure at the thought of sleeping all night bathed in that light.

"Then they shall take some of the blood and put it on the two doorposts and the lintel of the houses in which they eat them," said the Lord to Moses concerning the Passover. Years later when I read the story of the Exodus, I understood the source of the holy peace that filled my heart when my father marked the door of our house with the mark of the Passover Lamb.

"The blood of Christ, the cup of salvation." Forty years later, on my first Easter as a deacon, I was marking my brothers and sisters in Christ with the blood of that lamb. The angel of death would not touch them. I looked at my Lebanese friend, and I smiled back at him. *Christos Aneste. Alethos Aneste.*

Sometime in the next year I was standing again in white vestments on the chancel steps of the same church. Before me, under the bright white pall was the casket of my Lebanese friend. "Give rest, O Christ, to your servant with our saints . . ." Tears were burning in my eyes. I was not ready to give him up. Not yet. And then, in my soul's eye, I saw his smiling face turned up towards me at the altar rail again, and the faith he proclaimed to me that day, *Christos Aneste,* welled up within me. It was his gift to me to use for this moment. It was his faith that I was to proclaim today to the congregation. "*Alethos Aneste,* my friend," I whispered. And I looked up and said with conviction the beautiful and powerful words of the Commendation in the Book of Common Prayer, "All of us go down to the dust; yet even at the grave we make our song: Alleluia, alleluia, alleluia."

On the Way

The Very Rev. Durstan R. McDonald

It was a track and field meet, but not the ordinary kind. This one was special. There were races and the long jump, but also a softball throw in place of the shot put. This was the "Special Olympics."

One scene remains imprinted in my memory. It was a race to the finish line. The youngest runners were coming down their lanes, arms and legs akimbo, with broad smiles on their faces. Their gangly movements stood in vivid contrast to the sleek, powerful and well-coordinated Olympic athletes. But no matter. These racers were running, stumbling, and running again for all they were worth as the crowd of parents and friends cheered.

One runner raced with a crutch because one

side of his body was paralyzed. When he stumbled and fell, he got up again and continued the race. He and all the other racers were happy just to finish. Winning wasn't the issue for these children, but rather doing their best.

The atmosphere is completely different from the highly competitive, individualistic track and field races of ordinary Olympic athletes. They do not compete against one another, nor are they always comparing themselves to one another. They hug each other as they line up for a race. All the spectators cheer for each contestant. Can you think of a better image for our life as Christians?

Even now as the picture of these joyful, awkward athletes comes to mind, I find myself smiling. They've taught me something about what it means to be the Church.

Hines or Hogs?

The Rt. Rev. John E. Hines

I was born in the year 1910, in a small town in the Piedmont section of South Carolina. My father was a country doctor of remarkable breadth of vision and scientific acumen.

Later, and this may be an isolated phenomenon, it dawned upon me that the authentic priesthood being exercised in the religious economy of the town of Seneca lay with the medical profession in which my father exercised a ministry of integrity and humane concern, utterly selflessly for more than 50 years. He was, *de facto* if not *de jure*, the "high priest" of that community's spiritual life, officiating at their births, baptizing them into the real world of inescapable responsibilities, hearing their confessions (because he was the one unshakable center to whom they could repair in fair weather and foul and whom they trusted without reservation) and, finally, closing their eyelids in death. Countless were the children, white and black, who were named for him, so deep was their affection, so great their respect for him. His, indeed, may have been a priesthood after the order of Melchizedek which subsequent history appears to have authenticated.

In terms of authentic ministry, my father was also the town's prophet, although he would have been the first to disown any such status. Yet one story is illustrative of that unsought prophetic role. It had to do with the pitched battle he waged over a time-honored custom many townspeople had, of keeping their hog pens immediately adjacent to their homes. As the town's chief health officer, my father had been through more than one crisis, deriving directly from that hazardous proximity. Threatening the health of an entire community, the hog pens were a "time-bomb" ticking relentlessly away. So he approached the Town Fathers in solemn assembly and told them that the hog pens would have to be moved out of the town's municipal boundaries. The Town Fathers were polite (if stunned). They heard him out and, as is sometimes the case with political entities, did not do anything.

My father was a patient man, but he also was a very persistent man. After a period of quiet waiting, he returned to the town council and said, firmly, "Either the hogs go or I go!" That was serious, for he was the town's only health officer. If you had dropped an atomic bomb, you could not have caused greater consternation. They had to make a decision. So, reluctantly, they set a date for a vote, and the day before the vote, the town newspaper came out with headlines, "It's Hines or Hogs!" And, would you believe it, when the vote was taken, it was a tie. Three of the town councilmen voted for Hines, and three voted for hogs! But the mayor broke the tie: he voted for hogs, for the mayor owned the largest, most malodorous hog pen in town.

Well, it appeared that a pioneer had lost. The prophet had been rejected, but not for long. The epidemic my father foresaw came. And the mayor's only daughter contracted the disease and died. Soon after her funeral, the hog pens were removed from the town for grim catastrophe had succeeded where reasoned prophecy had failed. And the words of William Blake echoed thunderously through the streets of that chastened little town, "the tigers of wrath are wiser than the horses of instruction."

It was a daringly audacious thing that my father did. He listened to the drum beat of a different drummer from the one to whom his predecessors had listened.

He did it because he knew as a devout follower of Jesus Christ, that, Saint Augustine's famous oxymoron is still absolutely reliable for all Christians who wish to fulfill their prophetic vocation: "Love God, and do what you will."

Sister Mystica

The Rt. Rev. Furman Stough

I want to tell you about a woman I met in the Philippines some years ago. I went there with another priest to do some work for the Philippine Episcopal Church. Now, it helps to understand what is going on there with children if you understand something about the country. It is one of the poorest countries in Asia and perhaps in the world. Poverty is rampant throughout the Philippine Islands. A very small percentage of the people are extremely wealthy; the rest of them are just very poor. As in most countries of the world, poor people who live in the country believe that, if they can ever get to the city, things will be better—more medical help, better food, better education, jobs and so forth. As a result, Manila is overrun with literally thousands of quatters. Squatters' villages have been established all over that great metropolitan city. Some of these villages are huge. I saw one that contained 100,000 people and it was no larger than 40 acres.

There is no electricity, there is no running water, no sanitation facilities. You can imagine what happens—there is a great deal of sickness. The squatters also have a lot of babies, and if a baby appears to be in anyway sick or handicapped, it is usually abandoned. So in Manila you will find packs of young children running together. They scavenge, and do whatever they can to maintain their lives. They can be fierce; they even kill people. Some are no more than five or six years old.

The ministry that we wanted to see is conducted by a Roman Catholic order called the Missionary Sisters of Charity. That name may not mean anything to you, but I'm sure the name Mother Teresa does. This is her order. These sisters have established a home, an orphanage, for the children who are abandoned. The police and other people who know about this particular ministry bring them there.

It is located in the poorest part of old Manila. It is not a very large place, nothing is in that poor section. Ironically it is only a few blocks from the elegant presidential palace.

When we drove up, there were a lot of people gathered around, mostly women and children. They were holding a clinic. There is a great deal of respiratory disease in the Philippines today, and all of the children seem to cough most of the time. I looked at the medicine they were dispensing and most of it was over-the-counter remedies that you and I can buy in our drug stores. It won't cure those coughs, but simply help mask the symptoms and give them some temporary relief.

One thing you need to know about Mother Teresa's sisters is that they have one primary mission, no matter where they are and that is to help people die; to help poor people die with dignity. In Manila this ministry is to help babies and children die—those poor little ones who have been abandoned at some point along the way.

The sister in charge is named Mystica. She is one of the most stunning women I have ever seen, one of the most beautiful women I have ever seen. She has very dark skin, dark eyes, flashing beautiful white teeth and there is a radiance about her that is absolutely infectious.

She took us through one of the large areas where the babies are kept. It was a large room with nothing but rows of baby beds, one after another. Unfortunately, there are not enough sisters to do everything that needs to be done for these babies. People come in and help from time to time, but the most they can do is give the babies a little medicine to ease their pain, feed them, hold them as much as they can, and change their diapers. Being there is an overwhelming experience for someone like myself, born and raised in North America.

After we had gone through one building, we started towards another one and I said, "Sister, I don't believe that I can look at any more" and she smiled and said, "Why, of course, come let's have something to drink." We went out and sat down in the courtyard, and I said to her, "How long have you been here?" She said, "Nine years." I said, "How long have you been in charge?' "Seven years," she said. She was probably in her early thirties. I said, "Sister, I could not do what you do. I would be so devastated mentally, spiritually, emotionally, and physically that I could not do it. How do you do it?" And she looked at me with her wonderful smile and said, "Bishop, you don't understand. I have died with Christ. I no longer live. Christ lives in me and I can do whatever Christ wants me to do. My life is hid with God in Christ." And in my heart I thanked her for reminding me what it means to be a follower of Christ.

A Chance Meeting Stirs the Icy Heart

Eileen R. Suckley

I need glasses, so when I arrived at the library one morning at 9:00 only to discover that the sign said it opened at 9:30, I was totally exasperated. To make matters worse, there, seated on the marble doorstep, was the grubbiest street person I have ever encountered.

"Terrific," I thought. "My one morning of a dozen errands to run, and I'm going to waste thirty minutes of it with this derelict."

It was a hot, sultry morning without a hint of a breeze. I sat down at the farthest edge of the second step. The marble steps felt cool against my back. A cordon of ants marched their way along one of the cracks.

"See him?" my companion inquired.

"See whom?" I replied in my iciest tone.

"The muskrat," he said, pointing to the base of the tree on our right.

After a moment, "Yes, yes, I do see him!"

"He lives here . . . comes out every morning to collect his secret stash of food . . . third bush on the right."

"How do you know?"

"Because that's where I keep my stash."

"Why doesn't he eat yours, too?"

"Because mine is in a bottle with a cork stopper."

"Oh, I see."

"What's that?" he asked, pointing to my legal pad.

"It's my to-do list."

"Don't you know what to do without a list?"

"Yes, of course, well, no, I just . . . How do you keep *your* daily appointments in order?" I asked, making no effort to veil my sarcasm.

My companion just chuckled. "You never forget what's really important to you. What are you reading?" He pulled one of the books out of the top of my tote bag.

"Now, really," I began to sputter, but he interrupted, "T.S. Eliot—good man!"

"You read T.S. Eliot?" I asked incredulously.

"You know, you're a bit of a snob. Surely, the similarities between Prufrock and myself have not escaped you!"

"Not entirely."

"But I am most enamored of the *Four Quartets*: 'We shall not cease from exploration/ And the end of all our exploring/Will be to arrive where we started/And know the place for the first time.'"

I just sat there, off balance and uncomfortable. I absently wiped the sweat off the back of my neck. He reached into the recesses of his pocket and offered me a small flat bottle of some unspeakable libation. I did not avail myself of his hospitality, but it touched me. I knew he was offering what he had, all he had.

"No thanks."

He shrugged and started down the stairs to the street. "Wait!" I started down the steps after him. As he turned, I offered my hand across the space between us. "Goodbye, Mr. . . ."

"Winn," he replied, taking my hand and raising it to his lips. Then he bowed slightly and strode off. Cary Grant never made a smoother exit.

Almighty and everlasting God, who of his great mercy hath promised forgiveness of sins to all who with hearty repentance and true faith turn unto him, have mercy upon us—especially on one so blind of eye and callous of heart that she fails to see a child of God beaming in an unshaven face from the folds of a filthy overcoat.

I went back to the library several weeks later. The steps were empty. A landscaper was working in the front yard. The muskrat chose not to appear. I'd brought some cookies, wrapped tightly in foil. I placed them under the third bush on the right alongside a small bottle. It was No. 7 on my to-do list. Mr. Winn would have been amused.

It Wasn't One Of Ours!

The Rev. Richard H. Schmidt

You'd never mistake it for an Episcopal church.

It didn't look like a church, and Episcopal churches always look like churches! You could convert an Episcopal church into a hockey rink and it would still look like a church. But you had to keep reminding yourself this place was a church. It looked more like a bowling alley or hardware store, both of which it once was.

And the noises weren't Episcopal noises. I'm used to muffled sounds—kneelers thudding to the floor, overweight hymnals sliding into pew racks, soft-soled shoes shuffling along side aisles. But this place had abrupt noises.

The sermon was unlike anything heard from Episcopal pulpits. It resembled "Bolero" in that it began quietly but had you wanting to scream before it ended, which I thought it never would. It was about the dangers of alcohol and drug abuse by members of the congregation, a topic gingerly avoided by some Episcopal preachers in favor of more distant dangers like apartheid, the ozone layer and episcopal elections in other people's dioceses.

The prayers were gripping. Literally. The lady next to me gripped me when she implored the "Holy Ghost" to deliver her son from the evil the preacher had preached against. I didn't mind being gripped (though I didn't know whether to grip back) because I wanted to help this prayer along.

And of course, there wasn't any sacrament—or rather, there was the wrong sacrament, that is, not the one I wanted. The sacrament of unction was repeatedly celebrated, with laying on of hands and loud prayers for healing of the worshipers and their absent acquaintances. But there was no bread and wine so I felt sacramentally denied.

Then, when the service was over, several

people accosted me about coming to a Bible study after the service or to a prayer meeting that night. In some Episcopal churches, I might have been asked to sign the guest book, someone would have written me a note later in the week and that would have been that.

But the thing I'll remember most is the music. The music was awful. Most of it was in the Fanny J. Crosby style—lots of stuff about the blood of Jesus with the first person singular pronoun repeated over and over. The harmony consisted largely of three chords. But what really surprised me was that everyone sang. Loud. Lots of Episcopalians like to sing, too, but there are always some who use the hymn time to look at stained-glass windows and mumble to one another about the behavior of the acolytes. When several such Episcopalians congregate in the same pew, a lusty singer feels out of place.

I'm an Episcopalian who sings. Loud. That's one of the two reasons I go to church. The other is the sacrament—the one with the bread and wine. This hockey rink church may have lacked the sacrament, but the singing was riproaring. Though maudlin sentimentality isn't what I look for in a hymn, I'd rather sing blather in a roomful of other roof-raisers than feel self-concious doing a solo on David McK. Williams accompanied by the organist.

If forced to choose between the sacrament and singing, I'll take the sacrament every time. I want bread and wine on Sunday. That's why I'm an Episcopalian. But I may go visit that other church once in awhile, too. On account of the singing. And one or two other things.

Though Thank You's Are Seldom Heard

Dear Father Elwood:

This letter is long overdue, perhaps years overdue. I want to express to you, and to the entire family of St. Mark's Church, my appreciation and gratitude for the work of the church in the community. I deal with numerous churches of every kind throughout a fifteen county area, and I am pleased to say that none are more helpful or more compassionate in assisting those who, for a variety of reasons, can't always help themselves.

The outreach program of your church is enormous and wonderful. There are those who have no place else to turn, and so they turn to where Christian love is practiced daily, not simply preached, by those who know that one without the other is somehow not really complete.

I must tell you a true story about a mother with four little boys and a husband with tuberculosis. They were raised on welfare ($135.00 per month). They lived in Magnolia Gardens Housing Project for years. None of them were really expected to even finish high school, but they did. They all went to college, not without help, not without encouragement. One of those little boys became involved in a rewarding career, filled with meaningful work, and a deep appreciation for churches and the caring people who are indeed the church. By now you should know that the family I have described is my own family, and I am that little boy who was touched by the helping hands of others, others like the people of St. Mark's Church.

The people who make the work of St. Mark's Church possible may never really know when they have touched a life in a positive, loving way. Not everyone says "thank you;" not everyone will know how to express appreciation. But be assured that what you do is well worth the effort and it is a work worth being done. Please know that you and all the people of St. Mark's are appreciated much more than this letter can express.

Sincerely,

Armon Husband,
Human Services Specialist
Texas Department of
Human Services, Region 10

Summer Worship

The Rev. S. Albert Kennington

I love worshiping God in the Episcopal Church, especially in the summer as a visitor with my family.

Last Sunday I had such an opportunity in Christ Church, South Pittsburg, Tennessee. I worshiped with my family in a beautiful, old, white-frame, Gothic Revival house of prayer with dear friends on a lovely, sunny, summer morning. [With my loved ones around me, I sang the hymns, said "Amen" to the prayers, heard the Word, received our Lord at His table, and came away blessed.]

Between my car and the church porch I was welcomed warmly by men who sensibly left their coats at home and by women in cool summer dresses. Walking up the path, I thought to myself, "I know what's inside—old, dark wood, and organ music, and gleaming brass, an acolyte in victorious combat with a candlewick, the thud of a kneeler hitting the floor, the whispers of people not talking in church. Summer flowers would grace the retable. Up front the Bible would be open, and the table would be set with a place for me."

All was there as I expected, and more. My loved ones were not my only companions. I brought with me the problems of my week, my regrets and fears, the challenges waiting back home, my concerns for my flock, thoughts of a daughter soon to leave for college. All of me came to church. All of me is a lot for the church to handle.

The church was ready. The organ prelude ended as the procession bustled into formation. Familiar strains of an old hymn called us to our feet as a red-and-white-clad boy led the choir, carrying a brass cross almost too big for him. I sang about three words before the lump in my throat blocked the sound. The hymn was part of the church waiting for me, for all of me:

In the cross of Christ I glory,
towering o'er the wrecks of time;
all the light of sacred story
gathers round its head sublime.

This has never been one of my favorite hymns. The tune is cumbersome, the intervals a chore, the tempo always needing a boost. But I had forgotten the words:

When the woes of life o'ertake me,
hopes deceive, and fears annoy,
never shall the cross forsake me:
lo, it glows with peace and joy.

The young priest happily marked his first anniversary as Rector of the parish. He preached well from Galatians. During the Prayers of the People I silently remembered my own parish and our people offering the same worship at the same time.

After the Eucharist, lemonade and cookies were served on the lawn in the shade. Almost everyone stayed. (Imagine!) Children dressed for summertime played while grown-ups talked. The Episcopal Church is one big small town, and when viewed through the eyes of a summer Sunday worshiper, it is wonderful.

I do not worship on Sundays because I am good or because I am paid. I worship because I cannot live without it. I need to hear often that God loves me, that in Jesus Christ my sins are forgiven. I need to be strengthened in the Word and fed at the Table with my brothers and sisters around me. For these and all His mercies, I cannot keep from thanking Him and praising Him in the beauty of holiness and in the holiness of beauty. I am thankful without apology that I am a member of the Episcopal Church, especially on Sunday mornings.

Seeing the Angels Singing

The Rev. Weaver Stevens

Clergy, as is true with doctors and nurses, encounter the many shapes and surprises of God's unpredictable presence on the stage of life. Arthur Koestler, the novelist, once protested that God leaves the receiver off the hook, and this may be true if God is always dropping the phone to whip down here and make an unexpected entrance. I want to share with you one such unscheduled occurrence in which the fine hand of God might be suspected.

When a young curate at St. James, Wilshire Boulevard, I regularly took communion to the elderly "shut-ins" who lived in nearby apartments. Many were very lonely, having either no relatives, or relatives who paid little attention to them. They often had unique problems which were not seen by the social order flowing past their doors. I usually stopped for a cup of tea after administering communion, as this might be the only social call the elderly soul would receive for days on end. During one such "tea-stop" a little lady, named Ethel, hesitated and said, "I have a boy friend. Do you think that's all right?" "I think it's wonderful," I replied. "Even if we're sort of intimate?" "Especially, if you're sort of intimate." Her eyes were shining with tears. "We'd like you to come to supper at his place, some evening. Peter wants to meet you."

During the next year-and-a-half, I shared meals with them many times. We managed to develop a small network wherein this gentle couple entertained, visited, supported, and encouraged a good-sized circle of other, forgotten, elderly shut-ins. Then, Peter developed a serious flu which slipped into pneumonia. We had to take him to County Hospital where, due to a lack of facilities, he was placed with other elderly patients in a basement room of dreary dullness and great pipes running overhead. His system could not overcome the invasion and his condition became terminal.

During those last weeks, Ethel came down every day on the bus and sat for hours on a hard chair squeezed between his bed and a neighboring crib. Most of the patients were in cribs, with a constant crying, howling, shouting, cursing, pervading the over-crowded scene. This little lady never lost her sweetness, making friends, bringing small gifts with her on the bus, knitting booties, giving water, even giving sponge baths, as the nursing help was completely inadequate for such luxuries.

It was about a week before Christmas when Peter's last hours were at hand. I had commandeered another hard chair and was sitting near Ethel when Peter came out of his stupor and in a clear tone said, "Please sing some Christmas carols," and she did. Her unassuming, bell-like voice sailed lightly over the wailing sounds from the cribs. Soon a quiet ascended beneath her voice, then a few brave souls joined in timorously. A most unlikely choir was born. Somewhere along the way our friend died. She noticed, but kept singing. We didn't bother to call the nurse. Eventually one came in and made the expected fuss. I asked my little friend why she didn't cry. She laughed, "I guess you didn't see the angels singing with us. I did. And so did Peter."

As you might surmise, a major difficulty with God's stage appearances is that he often is not visible to a large segment of the audience. Even the Apostles had difficulty recognizing Jesus on the road to Emmaus.

Lunar Communion

Buzz Aldrin

On the day of the moon landing, we awoke at 5:30 a.m. Houston time. Neil and I separated from Mike Collins in the command module. Our powered descent was right on schedule. With only seconds worth of fuel left, we touched down at 3:30 p.m. . . . Now was the moment for Communion.

So I unstowed the elements in their flight packets. I put them and the Scripture reading in the little table in front of the abort guidance-system computer. Then I called back to Houston. "Houston, this is Eagle. This is LM Pilot speaking. I would like to request a few moments of silence. I would like to invite each person listening in, wherever and whomever they may be, to contemplate for a moment the events for the past few hours and give thanks in their own individual way."

For me, this meant taking Communion. In the blackout I opened the little plastic packages which contained bread and wine. I poured wine into the chalice my parish had given me. In the one-sixth gravity of the moon, the wine curled slowly and gracefully up the cup. It was interesting to think that the very first liquid ever poured on the moon and the first food eaten there were consecrated elements, the Body and Blood of Christ.

Just before I partook of the elements, I read the words which I had chosen to indicate our trust that as man probes into space, we are in fact acting in Christ. At that moment, I sensed especially strongly my unity with my church back home, and with the Church everywhere.

And Then There Are the Whales

The Rev. Chuck Meyer

The adventure was totally unexpected as most adventures are. It involved a boat on an unscheduled trip, twenty-five mentally impaired persons—and whales. My wife Debi and I were on vacation moseying around a fishing dock in Nova Scotia when a man in a pick-up asked if we were looking for a whale sighting cruise. We said we weren't but if he was going out we'd ride along. He was doing an unscheduled charter for a group and there might be enough room for two more—so we stuck around.

As they gathered, it was evident the people were from a local group home for the mentally retarded. Varying in age from 25-55, all were dressed for a boat trip with running-type shoes, jackets or sweaters, and sunglasses for the bright July sun. Some smoked nervously, others chewed gum or candy. There was much excitement at the prospect of seeing a whale. We got the last two seats on the side and greeted each other as the small boat plied its way through the blue water farther and farther off shore.

Debi was the first to sight the water spout, like a small geyser on the distant surface of the water, then another, and another. The captain nudged the boat of nervously elated people closer to the three humpbacks, until we were about 25 feet away.

These incredible creatures, three times the size of our boat, dove, cavorted, blew out their spouts, flapped their fins on the water, and showed the unique markings on the underside of their tails as they dove. All of us on the boat were spellbound, united in our awestruck sense of overwhelming size and grace and beauty.

And then the huge creatures stopped still in the water—and stared. Just below the surface they floated with eyes trained on the boat—or rather on the people in the boat. Like a scene from Star Trek or Cocoon, this boat full of persons of varying age and ability were staring eye-to-eye with three 70 foot sea creatures—and somehow communicating. Here there was no attempt to change one another, no judgment or demands, no better- or lesser-able. There was a sense of acceptance and affirmation that we were all one in that moment. And there was a peace on that sea that surely passed all understanding.

Somebody blinked—probably us—and the whales dove down under the boat, came up on the other side and flapped their fins as they swam away.

We all went back to our positions, chewed gum and smoked, waved at each other and tried to find other whales, but to no avail. Eventually we came back to shore and went our separate ways. But we were transformed by that encounter, reminded that there are more and older creatures here than we, reminded of our tiny place in the universe, yet affirmed and welcomed regardless of our ability or status.

If all of our daily interactions were that affirming and welcoming, we would have surely found the Kingdom of God. Perhaps it is enough to have seen a glimpse of it and to know it exists.

Real and Present Danger

Archbishop Michael Peers

Most of us are aware at some level or another that there is a crisis in the biosphere. We hear dramatic warnings from scientists about global warming, holes in the ozone layer, acid rain, the effects of pollution on lakes, rivers and oceans, the loss of the Amazon rain forests, PCBs and CFCs in the atmosphere. Certain new words have come into our vocabulary in the last few years, like Three Mile Island, Exxon Valdez, Chernobyl. My attention was first engaged in 1975 when a report by the Science Council of Canada put the whole matter in a visual image I could actually grasp:

"North Americans throw away enough

solid waste each year to build a wall 75 feet wide and 200 feet high along the Canada-US border."

Canadians grow up learning about our border with the U.S. as the longest undefended border in the world. The thought of an impenetrable pile of garbage stretching its entire length from just one year's refuse in our two countries is staggering. In the 16 years since the Science Council's report, the pile by now would extend all around the earth several times.

And yet, as we know, the environmental problem is about more than garbage. Recently there have been a series of highly publicized international conferences and commissions set up to look into the possible collapse of our global ecosystem. The best known of these is the Brundtland Commission of 1987. Here are some of its findings:

- every second an acre of forest is cut down
- every hour 1500 children die of hunger-related causes
- every week a species of life becomes extinct

- every year 20 billion tons of soil is eroded and lost

And yet there is hope, because some people are rediscovering the great mystical teachers of Christian tradition. As they go back in history, they discover saints and doctors of the church whose faith and vision of God never excluded the non-human world, nor ever imagined the human species to be the world's master. They call us back to this non-exploitative tradition, associated with names like Francis of Assisi and Julian of Norwich, with their concern for creation and the primacy of love.

These people have taught us about their spiritual traditions of harmony with God and respect for nature in ways that represent a fundamental critique of western theological tradition, with its emphasis on the superiority of human beings over other species, and its tendency to separate human life from nature's perpetual rhythms and seasons.

I have myself been instructed with great profit by Canadian aboriginal people as they have shown me some essentially negative and death-producing elements of western culture and how this has been undergirded by the church's denial of its own true sources of biblical revelation and teaching.

I recall vividly an incident when I was involved twenty years ago in the training of non-English-speaking Indian clergy in northern Ontario. One evening we were standing by a lake and saw a beaver swimming in the middle of the lake. One of the elders, Eliezer Beardy, called the beaver. The beaver stopped, turned, and swam to the shore and walked right to Eliezer who stooped down and stroked its head. Could I have done that? I thought not. Did Eliezer know something I didn't? I thought so then, and I think so now.

The Body of Christ

The Rt. Rev. Edward W. Jones

My first communion service was in a Presbyterian Church. I must have been twelve years of age because twelve in those days was the magical age when one was allowed to eat the bread and drink the wine, if you were an Episcopalian (if you were a Presbyterian, the bread and the grape juice). We didn't have goldfish wafers, we had little cubes of brown bread.

I recall that first communion because in those little pieces of bread and cups of grape juice I knew, somehow, I was in touch with something that was real and important in my life. Maybe at some point you have had that kind of experience too. That is about as near as I can come to explaining the words of Jesus when he said, "Truly, truly I say to you, unless you eat the flesh of man and drink his blood, you have no life in you. He who eats my flesh and drinks my blood has eternal life and I will raise him up at the last day." That's a truth even better known to the heart than to the mind.

Having earlier stepped on Presbyterian toes (lightly I trust), I now must tell a story about a Baptist gentleman who lived in a high-rise apartment building next door to a church I once served and who came to attend our services. When he came forward to receive communion, he would hold out his hands and I would put the bread in his hands. Then he would take the bread and put it in his pocket. He did that one Sunday and he did it a second Sunday. I began to harbor unkind thoughts— like, those Baptists know a lot about water but they don't know much about bread and wine. So I decided to go and see him and tell him how he ought to behave in church or something like that. I went up to his apartment and knocked on the door. He opened the door, I walked in and even before I spoke, he spoke and I understood. There in the room was his invalid wife and he began almost apologetically to say, "You may wonder why I take the bread and put it in my pocket each Sunday." And he said, "I do that so I may take it home and share it with my wife." That brief incident taught me a lesson I will never forget about the Eucharist and what it means to be the body of Christ.

A Christmas Basket

The Rev. Paul M. Washington

Every year on the Monday following Thanksgiving, Debbie, my secretary, asks, "Father, how many names should we take this year for the Christmas baskets?" I look up (which is my thinking pose) and pace the floor. Debbie smiles because she knows that at that moment I would not have means to promise even ten. Then I respond, "Let's plan for 250 families this year."

Usually, 250 families come in to sign up. Then "we wait on the Lord." As the days come and go, letters come in. "Dear Father Washington, here is a donation to help needy families at Christmas."

On December 20th we count the donations; there's always enough with fragments left over. Then we send letters to the families telling them to come to the church on December 24th to pick up their baskets.

Christmas Eve is busy and hectic. Volunteers pack baskets (bags) according to the size of the family, sometimes as many as ten per family. Then, at the given hour, the people come, present their letters and receive their gifts.

One year, one basket was unclaimed. We closed the office and prepared for the celebration of the 11 p.m. Christmas Eve service. After the servce was over we went home to get things ready for the family celebration and to get a little sleep.

Looking out of my stairwell window as I went upstairs I saw that I had left the lights on in one of our church buildings. I decided (I don't know why) to go back to the church to turn off the lights. It was about 2 a.m. As I approached the gate, I saw a woman standing there.

I said, "Good morning. Merry Christmas."

She took a letter from her pocket and said,

"I was supposed to get a Christmas basket today, but somebody else in my house got the letter and just gave it to me a little while ago. Can I still get my basket?" I looked at her with a smile of astonishment and utter disbelief. I said, "Lady, did you really expect to find somebody here at two o'clock in the morning?"

She was embarrassed. In asking her that question, I had humiliated her.

For, in a sense, I was asking, are you so poor and desperate and maybe so dumb that you would come to church on this cold winter night at such an hour for a Christmas basket?

But like the Samaritan woman who totally disarmed Jesus when she said, "Yes, Master, but even the dogs eat the crumbs that fall from the master's table" (Matthew 15:27), she simply responded, "I don't know, sir, but I thought I would try."

I said, "Lady, God bless you. You have a lot of faith. Your basket is here."

She came into the parish house with me. I gave it to her and wished her and her children a Merry Christmas.

Accepting the basket, she wished me a Merry Christmas and disappeared into that silent, Holy Night. May God bless you all this Christmastide.

Lewis Green's Class

The Rev. Stephen Stanley

When I was ten years old, I was "recruited" into Lewis Green's Sunday school class. I say "recruited" because Lewis was an ex-marine drill sergeant turned newspaper reporter and Sunday school teacher.

My older brother and some of his friends had preceded me in this venture, and their activities were a source of wonder to me, fueling my desire to belong. It was my brother's friend who finally convinced both my brother and Lewis that this skinny little kid had the makings of a raw recruit. Thus, I became a life-long member of the church school regiment that called itself the Unsophisticated Meatballs.

I was given the rank of buck private and told that there were expectations on my life which, if adhered to, would result in my rising through the ranks in due time.

The "Unsophisticated Meatballs" met on Sunday morning as did other classes, and did some typical things like Bible study and singing. However, I cannot remember any of the specifics of what we learned in those class sessions. But I do remember that Lewis ran a tight ship.

Even more memorable were the frequent camping trips to Lewis's favorite wilderness, a place called Wild Cat Cliffs. Lewis was also a great storyteller, and I can remember sitting around the campfire on dark nights at Wild Cat Cliffs, being scared out of my wits by stories like "The Ghost Who Lost His Golden Leg." Some of our camping trips were all weekend affairs which, I remember, caused a lot of conflict in the parish. "Why aren't the kids in church this Sunday?" was one refrain.

Lewis was not too popular with the more traditional Sunday school teachers, but I recall that the more abuse he suffered, the more we all rallied to his cause.

Over the course of four years I rose in the

ranks to technical sergeant, and received several printed certificates saying that the following person had been "declared an Unsophisticated Meatball in good standing and has achieved the rank of . . . on this day . . . "

I've long since forgotten what Lewis Green taught me about religion, but I've never forgotten that I belonged to a special community, and grew in my identity through that experience. It was my first experience of church fellowship in which I was given a Name and Purpose. There was preparation for the future, there was an experience of common growth in the Gospel, although I would not have named it so at the time (and many others would not have either).

Full awareness of my growth came more than twenty years after my graduation from that class. I ran into another Meatball whom I had not seen since childhood. He remembered, and he said there were others who had never forgotten either.

▼▲▼

Jenny

The Very Rev. Walter H. Taylor

One of the cherished memories of my first years as a priest is that of a woman named Jenny. She was well into her eighties when I first met her. Never married, she lived alone in a small apartment that was modest by anyone's standards. Although she was still alert and full of life, she had difficulty walking, so generally she stayed close to home where she entertained a group of friends whose number grew smaller each year.

The first time I visited Jenny I had at my fingertips, so I believed, all the pastoral insights and techniques I would ever need. We had a pleasant visit and shared some coffee at her kitchen table, and when I got up to leave, I asked her whether she would like to have a prayer together. Without a moment's hesitation she was cheerfully kneeling on the linoleum floor, and before I could say a word, she started to pray. I don't remember her exact words, but it was a simple prayer offered for the young clergyman kneeling beside her.

Almost thirty years later, I still feel warmed by the memory of Jenny and her prayer. I remember feeling surprised initially that she was the one praying. After all, everyone knows that it is the clergy who are supposed to do that! I was also touched that this dear, old woman with so many problems of her own was more concerned about me than about herself.

That afternoon Jenny taught me some important lessons. By her example she under- scored that we are all called—clergy and laity alike—to minister to one another. Clergy do not have a corner on the faith and tranquillity market. In fact, we very much need the prayers and caring support of lay persons day by day. As someone once pointed out, beware of those clergy who always seem to have life and limb joyfully and seamlessly together, because they are the ones who usually don't.

Perhaps even more importantly, Jenny demonstrated profoundly but simply that when we become more concerned about others than we are about ourselves, the frustrations and burdens of life are somehow easier to bear or, as in Jenny's case, seem to exist not at all.